Chapters

I0447222

Chapter 1 – What the hypnotist is and is not

"Watch the swinging watch. See how it goes. Left and right, right and left. As it swings, left and right, notice how your eyelids are getting heavier and heavier until you cannot keep them open any longer. You are falling deeply asleep. Deeply asleep. You are falling into my power. Your thoughts are now mine and my words are your deeds. "

If this is how you think of hypnosis then you have seen one too many movies and your image of a hypnotist is probably one of a dark-haired figure with a goatee beard and a monotone voice, about to enslave a young woman to his evil will or to entice a man to commit murder. It is this image that makes the hypnotist a caricature of the wicked villain and makes you fearful of the power he could hold over you.

This one myth is probably responsible for more people shunning hypnosis and denying themselves relief from a huge number of mental and physical problems. If this book does nothing more than dispelling that representation of the hypnotist then I will consider that it has done a good job. Of course I want to do much more for you and over the remaining pages I will do my best to make you aware of what hypnosis can (and can't) do for you, but can only do so when you are ready and have a mind to co-operate with the hypnotist.

First of all, your average modern-day hypnotist seldom uses the swinging watch technique (and if he does it will more likely be backwards and forwards rather than left and right). If this is disappointing to you and you expect it when you visit the hypnotist, then make sure you tell him (or her). Good hypnotists want to work with you and within your beliefs. It makes their job so much easier then trying to bend you to theirs. Of course, the first time you visit a hypnotist they will probably give you a little talk before they start (or ask you to watch a video or listen to a recording), which explains a little of what they do and what you can expect, and the really good ones will give you a chance to ask questions before they start. After this pre-talk, your new understanding of the hypnotic process will lead to better co-operation from you and better results for you too. In general though, your expectations are the ones that need to be met and as you are paying the bill, you should have a say in how you are hypnotised. You are the one paying the piper, you should call the tune.

Another thing that may disappoint you about the hypnotist is how normal they look. A dark beard is not a pre-requisite (especially for the female hypnotists), nor are hooded eyes or a monotone voice pattern a requirement. Most are not medically, psychiatrically or otherwise professionally qualified (in some countries though, they have to be) so don't be surprised if the hypnotist requests you get medical referrals before they continue. Your hypnotist will want to make sure that they are not treading on some other professional's toes before treating you for a problem.

You may see some certificates on the wall and chances are they will be from various hypnosis organisations stating courses attended or memberships of local, national or international organisations. Take heart from these, especially if they have a spread of dates. They show that the hypnotist is willing to spend money on keeping himself trained and aware of different ideas. New techniques and thoughts appear regularly in all worlds and hypnosis is no different in that respect. The hypnotist who at least checks out different opinions will be a better therapist for it, even if the ideas are not liked by him or her.

So what else can you expect from your new friend, the hypnotist? Probably the same as you would expect from any therapist - the willingness to listen to you, after all – you are the one who knows what you are there for, the ability to advise whether he can help you and to do so to the best of his abilities. The hypnotist will then be able to adapt the way you are dealt with in accordance with your wishes thus helping to believe more fully in the results you both want achieved.

The more astute of you will notice that I have not used the word 'hypnotherapist' yet. Although it is an accurate term for a therapist who uses hypnosis, I personally am against the idea of separating hypnosis for therapy from hypnosis for entertainment (stage hypnosis or street hypnosis). This is because apart from what is done under hypnosis (the intent), there is little to no difference between them. The same techniques of how to get someone into hypnosis would mostly work in the different settings although the appreciation for the 'how' may be seen very differently. The long relaxation technique often used in therapy sessions would not be exciting to watch in an entertainment setting, nor would the dramatic 'instant or rapid' hypnotic induction usually be appropriate in the calm atmosphere of the therapy session. There are exceptions, as some of my fellow hypnotists would be quick to point out, but it is better to learn the rules first so the exceptions can then be appreciated and possibly used when necessary.

So you now have a good idea of what a hypnotist is and isn't. We will now go on to what hypnosis is (and isn't). What it is good for and we'll go deeper and deeper (hypnotist's joke) into how hypnosis can help you, not only with smoking, dieting and phobias (the main problems that hypnosis is asked to help with) but with larger and smaller things too. When self-hypnosis is a good idea and when it's not and some things you might like to ask of your hypnotist before they start on you.

Chapter 2 – What you need to know about hypnosis

The first big revelation is hypnosis is not sleep. When you're asleep you are probably the world's worst conversationalist. You are aware of very little that goes on around you and you're certainly not lucid enough to answer questions or take in ideas being given to you. Under hypnosis you are hyper-aware, far more than you are in your 'normal waking' state. Your conscious 'here and now' mind can only deal with 5 to 9 pieces of information at a time (try remembering a list of 10 - 12 items without grouping them or using mnemonic techniques) whereas your unconscious mind can cope with much more and has processing power to spare to listen to that far away siren or the deeper meanings of the words that are being spoken to you. It is this unconscious mind that is brought to the forefront when you are hypnotised, and your conscious mind that is given a short break.

Think of something familiar to you, like your home phone number. Where was that number just before you thought of it? Not in your immediate memory because you didn't need it until I asked you to think of it, but as soon as you were reminded of it, it popped up for you from your unconscious mind. You have conditioned your mind to keep that piece of information handy but you don't need it 24/7 so it doesn't stay consciously ready for action.

Hypnotic trance is a natural phenomenon. You've experienced hypnotic type effects every day of your life. Just before going to sleep and just before becoming fully awake, daydreaming or drifting your mind whilst engaged on a routine task are examples of this. You're not consciously concentrating on the task in hand, although if something unusual occurred your focus would snap to the task, like if you're driving on a routine journey you can listen to the radio and sing along to a favourite song quite happily, aware of the traffic around you but not letting it affect you or your progress, until someone cuts you up a little finer than you'd like and suddenly the singing stops and all your concentration is on your driving and involved in keeping you safe.

Much of the unconscious mind is involved in that one last fact, keeping you safe. If you accidentally touch a hot surface, you will pull away without a second thought. The blare of a car horn whilst you are crossing the road will have your feet running from its source before your brain has time to think "speed up" and you will generally duck or at least flinch without thinking if you hear a loud noise. All actions designed with your well-being in mind. This is something your unconscious mind is good at and having this one thought in your head when you visit a hypnotist will give you far more confidence whilst you are under hypnosis, because your unconscious mind will keep you safe. Safe from physical harm – your unconscious mind will reject a situation that would harm you or that you need to react to – say a fire alarm going off, and safe from mental harm – your mind would reject an unsafe or embarrassing suggestion as not good for you.

Sometimes your conscious mind gets in the way of the good running of your body and life.

Let's make an easy to understand simile of this:

Imagine a well run cruise ship. The captain is in charge and so long as he stays on the bridge, checking his charts and directing where the ship will go, all is well.

Now imagine what would happen if the captain decided not to trust the crew and he now wants to cook the meals, lay the tables, serve the guests, check the engines, do everybody's laundry, organise the entertainment, in short he tries to micro-manage every function of the running of all of looking after the guests and the thousands of other things that happen on this previously well run ship. Who then is watching where the ship goes?

The captain is your conscious mind and it is good a 'big picture', over all stuff, whilst your unconscious mind deals with the routine stuff, like breathing, heartbeat, what the spleen does, regulating your body temperature within life sustaining margins and all those other things that you help to keep you yourself fit and healthy. On the occasions that your conscious mind tries to take over some aspect of what should be an unconscious activity; things can sometimes go wrong, sometimes very wrong and this is when hypnosis can come in, push the conscious mind back to its proper job of overseeing without interfering.

A phobia is probably the best example of this. If you have a fear of flying you constantly consciously think of all the things that could go wrong with the aircraft, the pilots or the crew. Logically (unconsciously) you know that there are thousands of flights every day, all over the world that are totally without any sort of mishap, the pilots are well trained and the cabin crew know how to do far more than bring you drinks with a smile, but your conscious mind concentrates on all the bad things that could happen although they seldom do. Hypnotically you and the hypnotist (it's a joint effort) would then put those fears back into their proper perspective and guide your conscious mind back into thinking something more suitable for whilst you are flying. The phobic person may not ever love flying (although that is possible) but they will always be comfortable or even nonchalant about the idea.

This is a good time to dispel a few misconceptions about hypnosis as many of them come back to the statement made in a previous paragraph about your unconscious mind keeping you safe from internal and external harm.

You cannot get 'stuck' in hypnosis. This widely held myth probably comes from the days when travelling hypnotists would do what is known as the 'Store Window Stunt' where, along with a poster advertising the stage hypnotist's show in a local theatre in the next week, there would be a young lady asleep in a bed with a card beside her, stating she would stay there, asleep, until just before the show, when the hypnotist would awaken her. In reality the young lady would be awakened for a few hours in the dead of each night to allow her to be fed and get some exercise before being hypnotised again to sleep through the next day. However, the illusion that she was asleep all the while because of hypnosis is possibly the basis of the idea that people could stay stuck in hypnosis for a long time.

This idea of being stuck could also be related to the fear of something happening to the hypnotist whilst his volunteers were in a trance and them not being able to wake up from it. Exactly like the sudden lack of noise in any situation, that background hum that disappears and brings itself to your attention, the incessant conversationalist who decides to (finally) stop speaking. The lack is apparent by its very absence and so it is if the hypnotist goes silent for too long for any reason. The hypnotee would gradually come out of their trance and wonder why it's gone so quiet all of a sudden.

A recent publicity stunt was done by a British stage hypnotist during which, he hypnotised a group of college students and then fell off the stage, allegedly knocking himself unconscious. The news report claimed his volunteers were safe because he had left a tape to be played in the eventuality he was not available to awaken them in person. He was lambasted by his hypnosis peers for making out there was a danger where none really existed as he implied the volunteers would not come out of trance without him. In reality the tape would not have been required as the students would have come out of the hypnotic trance in their own good time.

You cannot be forced to do anything you wouldn't normally do. Alright, I'll admit there's a bit of debate on this one in that some clever wording and some knowledge of your own mind and habits could possibly make you do a few things that you wouldn't do whilst fully awake, very much like you may sing and dance energetically if you get too drunk, but there are so many 'maybes' and 'if onlys' that it would be difficult even for a highly hypnotist. Your mind and morals have been together for a long time and if they feel that something is not quite right with what the hypnotist is saying then it is more than likely that you will reject the hypnotist's suggestion and you will come out of trance. You know, and it's deeply ingrained in you, that you try your best to keep your passwords secret so it is unlikely that you would tell them to anyone who asks, even under hypnosis.

"Ah", you say. "But what about those volunteers on stage? You can't tell me they want to act like chickens or dance like Madonna?" Well actually, they do. A stage hypnotist is looking for exhibitionists when his show starts as they are easier to work with (up to a point!). They, not the hypnotist, are the stars of the show. They want people to look at them. In other words, they have an excuse to do what they are told to be the centre of attention (and not take the blame... "The hypnotist told me to do it") and a good thing too. Without them, there is no show! However, if you're watching a show that is still doing chicken impersonations or dancing like Madonna when 'Like A Virgin' is played, it's probably time the hypnotist updated his act. Modern stage hypnotists have to put more imagination into their shows these days. The public expects more and one of the first rules of hypnosis is 'go with what the public expects'.

Surprisingly though, you can lie under hypnosis, especially if it something you could normally not tell the truth over, and even hypnosis could not normally force you to tell the truth. Of course, if you are an immoral person, someone who would readily steal something or harm someone then it would be easier (not necessarily very easy) to make you do so under hypnosis as you are not really going against your 'waking' inclinations. Such a person would probably lie if questioned under normal circumstances and could easily do so when in trance, but having said that, most of us can lie for the right reasons and this ability does not go away just because we are in hypnosis. I make no comments on this point about hypnotising estate agents, politicians or lawyers and still expecting straight or honest answers!

In relation to lying under hypnosis we can also omit something we've been asked, if we feel uncomfortable with the question or the outcomes of its answer, so if the hypnotist (or anyone around them) asks "Have you ever been unfaithful to your partner", it is likely that the recipient of the question might refuse to answer. A good hypnotist will cover himself from anyone else asking awkward questions by stating during the hypnotic process that the volunteer will only hear his instructions. This avoids someone else trying to make use of the rapport and trance that the hypnotist has got with the volunteer.

Hypnosis is very much a collaborative process between hypnotist and hypnotee, and the hypnotist who asks stupid, awkward or uncomfortable questions is very likely to lose the most important thing that they had with their victim and that is their trust. As stage or therapy hypnotists we spend much of our initial time gaining the trust of our volunteers and clients and it is this rapport that could be ruined so easily with bad questions or poor technique, especially if you came to us asking for help with a phobia or something sensitive or personal. One poorly voiced question or statement could destroy any good work we may have done gaining that rapport and wreck any chance of assisting the patient to an effective cure for their problem or the volunteer from putting on a great show for the audience.

One last myth is that only the weak willed can be hypnotised and repeated hypnosis makes the will even weaker. In fact the opposite is true on both counts. A strong willed person usually makes an excellent hypnotic subject especially when it comes to 'mind improvement' changes. You would not accuse a professional sportsman or a top businessman of being weak willed but these are the type of people who benefit from ego-strengthening mental exercises or good-habit ingraining to improve their performances even further. What's more, through the repetition of the hypnotic process, it does make it easier to go back into hypnosis, the trance usually gets deeper with the repetitions and both the hypnotist and the client get more satisfactory work done and usually in a shorter time, though this does not mean the client is losing his will to the hypnotist, just that the trust and rapport is already established and both know and trust the other, and with that established, the results will be even more pronounced.

As a final point, and this applies more to entertainment hypnosis (which tends to be a bit more active), you should not volunteer to be hypnotised if you are drunk or drugged, (since you think you are hypnotised already), if you are pregnant (but only since there may be some physical activity. Not because hypnosis is dangerous to a pregnant woman) or if you suffer from any sort of unusual mental disorders, especially epilepsy or the like. There is a small likelihood of triggering an episode that will not look good for you or the hypnotist. Even in a therapy situation the hypnotist should ensure that you do not fall into these categories and only trained specialists should be trying to treat mental disorders with hypnotism. Hypno-birthing, a technique used to reduce the labour pains, should only be considered after consulting with maternity professionals.

Chapter 3 - Rapport and Trust

I've mentioned these two words several times in the previous chapter, but what do they actually mean, on the face side of the swinging watch?

The latter word is easy. It means that you trust the hypnotist, to do what you came to him for and in such a way that you will feel good about the change being affected on you, whether in the therapy room or on stage. It also means that the hypnotist trusts you! Read that bit again... **The hypnotist must also trust you**. He trusts that you came into the situation with honest intentions as to the outcome, because if you didn't there is no point in either of you being there.

Notice that I haven't said that the hypnotist trusts you to go into a trance. If you merely 'played along' and pretended to go into a trance, chances are the outcome would still be what you wanted. Why? Because you still trusted the hypnotist enough to go along with what he was saying. It doesn't matter that your conscious mind wasn't 'away with the fairies' or whatever you expected to happen whilst your unconscious mind was having some aims redirected. All that matters is that the two way trust was established between you both. How that trust was gained is the topic of the first word of the title of this chapter... Rapport.

With a good hypnotist (and I'm sorry to say there are some out there who are not as good as they could be, and as is usual in human nature, there are some who shouldn't even be hypnotists at all), probably more effort is spent on rapport building with each client than is passed with hypnosis. Rapport is the building block of being able to do change work under hypnosis. It ought to begin with a simple "Hello", an introduction, a small beginning that should end up with the total trust necessary for the hypnotic work to commence, but in reality it could begin before even that.

In the hypnotist's office, there are probably some certificates on the wall, nicely framed and proudly proclaiming that the hypnotist has done this course or that or is a member of a national or international group of hypnotists. Look at all those posh bits of paper. This guy must know his stuff.

On stage, you might not get to see the bits of paper, but you will have seen the posters proudly proclaiming the world's greatest hypnotist (funny that he's never the 2nd greatest or maybe further down the pecking order), you've read reviews of other performances in the press or on the internet or maybe heard an interview on the radio and possibly hypnotising the presenter or his assistant. Before the audience is invited up on stage (or sometimes afterwards, depending on how the hypnotist runs his shows) there will have been some exercises, games or tests of suggestibility that the hypnotist will have run through to see if any of the audience would make good hypnotic subjects. These all amount to the same thing as those certificates.

In whatever situation 'The Hypnotist' (note the capitals, every hypnotist is always THE Hypnotist) will greet you with confidence. Somebody who knows what they're doing, has belief in their own abilities must be the 'real deal'. You can't fail to be on a winner. He speaks clearly and concisely to you, answers your questions without hesitation. He must be good! He is someone you can work with (not 'for'. Hypnosis remember, is a partnership).

If trust is the required end result and rapport is the primary building block of that trust, then the secondary building block is intent. The intent to be put on the road to recovery from whatever problem you came in with. The intent is for you to lose weight or to give up smoking, if one of those is your desire. The intent is for you to have a good time and to be the star of the show, if you're on stage.

The hypnotist's intent is to help the client to achieve his goals, and it is this partnership between the hypnotist and the client, brought on by rapport and trust that will turn intent into achievement.

Chapter 4 - So What Happens Next?

Is it time for the swinging watch yet? As I said in chapter 1, the chances are that you won't see a watch at all, least not a swinging one unless you really, sincerely, strongly believe that you can't be hypnotised without one.

Initially you may be asked to do some exercises or tests or hypnotic-like demonstrations, whatever the hypnotist would like to call them, as a means of showing you the power of the hypnotist's words. These are not 'pass or fail' tests as such, nor are they hypnosis in any deep sense of the word. They are merely guidelines for the hypnotist and yourself that prove you can listen and follow simple instructions.

There are many of these exercises and here are some examples:

- The locked arm, where you are led to believe that you cannot bend your arm.
- Light / Heavy hands, where one hand is piled high with imaginary heavy books and the other with an accumulation of helium balloons.
- Stuck hand – your hand is stuck to a table, wall or a part of your body.
- Locked fingers, which is when the hypnotist tells you your hands are stuck together and you cannot separate them.

There are many other ideas but these are the most commonly used ones. Sometimes these exercises may be the introduction to the induction into trance, but usually they are just there to get the party started.

Once these exercises are complete we may then get more into an actual induction into hypnosis although to be honest, almost everything the hypnotist has said and done up to this point has been part of the initial preparation for hypnosis. You have been convinced the hypnotist knows his stuff and he is convinced that you believe it all too.

And now for the actual hypnotic induction as you might recognise it...

You may be asked to stare into a light or at a spot on the wall or even a spinning disk with a spiral pattern on it or even the palm of your hand. None of these are strictly necessary and all each of these things has in common is that they are a distraction for your conscious mind so that the hypnotist can get in touch with your unconscious mind – the entity who really controls the 'self' who you are. This is the beginning of an induction.

The hypnotist will probably be speaking to you in a quiet clear voice, usually quite slowly and you may be surprised to learn that you may go into a trance more because of boredom than anything else. This is intentional in the beginning although if you become a regular to the same hypnotist you may be introduced to something known as a 'rapid induction' since you keep coming back, you must have a lot of trust and faith in the hypnotist. Everything, at least in a therapy situation will be done in slow time and with your comfort and well being in mind.

On stage the process may be similar but the volume and pace may be a bit different. The stage hypnotist wants the audience to know what's going on and how in control he is. He wants you to know that too, and he wants it to happen quicker than it would in a therapy situation. Twenty minutes spent getting you under might be fine in the office, but it's boring to watch on stage, so you may well see an instant or shock induction being performed here. The end result is the same though whether you are bored into a trance or shocked into it, your conscious mind is being distracted so your unconscious mind can take over for a while.

I will add at this point that a shock induction is not painful nor is it all that shocking. If it is, then the entertainer is doing it wrong and could be causing injury and this may be a good time to 'wake up' and get away from him, or at least check his liability insurance is paid up and valid.

I could at this point tell you the words that the hypnotist will be using, but there are as many forms of the wording as there are hypnotists. There should be some light animation in the hypnotist's voice. Anyone who thinks a monotone is necessary is either reading off a prepared script (which the hypnotist himself may not have prepared) or has an old-fashioned approach to hypnosis. The wording will include references to relaxing and the eyes closing but don't expect to be asleep by the end of it. As I said in the beginning, sleeping people are terrible conversationalists!

How will you know when you're in a trance? Well you might know or you might not. You may just be thinking to yourself, "I wonder when something is going to happen" just as you're being told to be back in the room or you may be aware of every word the hypnotist says. It really doesn't matter as long as you feel you are in a position to accept the hypnotist's suggestions, and you're doing that because you have rapport with him and you trust him implicitly.

It is at this point that just as you're settling nicely into a trance-like state the hypnotist may tell you to open your eyes and then close them again. He's not being awkward, he's just re-hypnotising you and helping your mind to get used to the idea using the process known as 'fractionation'. Remember I said before about hypnotising being easier for you the more times it happens to you? Well research has shown that the time period between hypnosis sessions doesn't have to be months, weeks, days or even hours. A second or so is enough. This is why in the stage setting, the skits performed by the volunteers get progressively more involved as the show goes on. They are getting more used to being hypnotised and so go easier and deeper into trance each time and the trust they have in the hypnotist is also improved since they hear his praise and the audience's applause (which is what they really want).

Another thing that the hypnotist should do somewhere along the line once you are in your trance state are those little exercises I mentioned previously, only now they are known as 'convincers', since they convince you that you are definitely hypnotised.

The clever hypnotist also knows that the public thinks that amnesia is a feature of hypnosis (especially since he might have suggested it earlier in his pre-hypnosis speech) and will suggest to you to forget certain parts or even all of the induction or the trance just so you will 'know' that you have been hypnotised.

Will knowing all of these things actually prevent you from being hypnotised? In a word – no, otherwise you could never hypnotise a hypnotist and many of them actually make very good hypnotic subjects. Not wanting to be hypnotised will make it more difficult for the hypnotist but knowing the process won't. In fact it should make it easier if you know what's going on and what is likely to happen next. There are hypno-junkies who will quite happily be hypnotised at the drop of a hat and they probably will already know as much about hypnosis as they can possibly find out.

Talking of being hypnotised at the drop of a hat is a good time to go back to rapid, instant and shock inductions, what each of them is and when they might be successfully used.

A rapid induction is used by both the stage and office hypnotist, usually on someone who has been hypnotised before and therefore knows what is expected of them. It is set up by the hypnotist for use on a future occasion (even if that is only a few seconds or minutes into the future) and consists of a hypnotic suggestion to go back into a trance on a specific signal – Much like when a stage hypnotist place a hand on the shoulder of an individual and says "sleep". In a stage show this is done many times and quickly becomes a habit for the volunteer and enables the hypnotist to keep control over his panel and also impresses the audience too with his total control over his subjects.

The danger that a non-hypnotist might make use of this trigger action for their own purposes can be eliminated by the hypnotist specifying that only he, and only for the purposes of hypnosis, can activate the trigger signal or it can only take place in his office or on this stage and the suggestion cannot be activated once the client has left the location.

An instant or shock induction is also brought about by a trigger action, but this time it is not pre-induced. Some street hypnotists use an almost violent pull forward of the body during a handshake to cause a shock but this is considered dangerous by many as the hypnotist may not know in advance whether the intended victim has a back or neck problem which could be made worse by such an action. It is usually enough just to change the pattern of a handshake or reach behind a person's neck to tip the head forward and say in a commanding voice 'sleep' (no need to shout) to distract attention rather than shock the conscious mind into submission. It is still almost necessary to know that the person performing this type of induction is a hypnotist and that hypnotism is expected. After all, someone shouting sleep at you is hardly likely to induce you into a hypnotic trance if you didn't know that was what they (and you) wanted.

So once you're in trance, will you behave like a mindless zombie and become the hypno-slave of the hypnotist? Well if you've been following the contents of this book, you'll already know that the answer is 'no'. You will retain an element of your own will and morals although you will be more open to suggestions as to your behaviour and you will be in a position to accept new ideas to help change your life, whether for your own benefit or for the entertainment of yourself and others.

What about the 'other end' of hypnosis? What happens when you finished being the world's greatest entertainer (under the direction of the hypnotist) or you have had your treatment for smoking, weight-loss or phobia? How will you be 'emerged' from this deep and wonderful trance?

As it is for getting you into a trance, there are various techniques for getting you out again, some good and some not-so-good.

The less than optimal hypnotist will just get you to wake up and tell you that you are back in the room, then send you on your way. This has little concern for your well-being and is also missing a few things that could make a lot of difference to you.

A better hypnotist will bring you back a little more gradually, counting up, putting more animation into his voice and tell you that you feel great, that your head is clear and that the world is a wonderful place for you to be in.

The best hypnotists will never ask you "How do you feel?" after they have brought you out of your trance. They'll tell you that you feel really good, that any lingering stiffness is fading away, and even after they tell you "eyes open, wide awake" (or whatever their chosen message), they will carry on giving you reinforcing and positive messages as they know you will still be receptive to suggestions for a few more minutes yet.

In a therapy situation, this is a good time to have a glass of water as some of the physiological effects may have had-flushed face or raised body temperature, and having a few sips of water will help cool you down and rehydrate you. Chances are if you've just been on stage then someone will be offering you a drink anyway. Alcohol is not the ideal refreshment in this situation but it will be some fluid to help your body a bit. Ask for fruit juice or water for now and your body will thank you for it later.

Chapter 5 – So what is hypnosis good for?

I've mentioned a few times the most common requests for hypnosis treatment – to help quit smoking, to help with weight loss and to remove phobias. What other things can be treated with hypnosis and to what other uses can hypnosis be put to as an aid to daily living?

I did a search for this on the internet and found someone had put up a list of over a hundred things that hypnosis can help with. The list can be condensed down into a few categories:-

Eliminate bad habits (smoking, over-eating, nail biting)

Pain relief (Irritable Bowel Syndrome, point anaesthesia, dental or pregnancy pains)

Enhance good habits (exercise, positive thinking)

Performance enhancement (improve your golf, sexual activity)

Relaxation (Stress relief)

Entertainment (Stage hypnosis, past life regression)

Although the list is not exhaustive it should give an idea of what can be treated or assisted by hypnosis. If you have an idea, approach your hypnotist with it. They should be receptive and have an idea of how to proceed with helping you. The biggest help you can give your hypnotist is that he

CAN help you. A positive mindset is by far the best step forward for you.

I have one important note of advice here. Hypnosis can, if done properly, usually totally eliminate pain, but this is seldom a good thing. How about if you went to a hypnotist and said you had run into a door and had a pain in your chest that you were sure was just a painful bruise and could he take the pain away. You're sure the pain is related to your accident and taking it away will help you cope for now. The pain actually turns out to be a broken rib or you have a heart attack which you don't know about because you've had the pain 'switched off' in that area. A good hypnotist will raise these points with you and will be able to reduce your pain to more tolerable levels for you, but will seldom eliminate the pain totally even when he could. This is for your protection as much as his and is to ensure you seek proper medical help if the need arises.

Glove (Point) Anaesthesia is an interesting technique where the ability and responsibility is given to the person who needs it. They are told (under hypnosis, of course) that when they concentrate, that their hand has a temporary anaesthetic effect on any part of their own body it touches. This allows them to numb pain in a localised area for a short time while under their own control, which can be important for some people. It often seems bad enough that you hand over control to a hypnotist, even when you know it will be of benefit to you. If can take back or retain some control, the effective results for you could be so much better.

As serious a subject as it can be for some people, Past Life Regression has to be put in the 'entertainment' category, at least in the UK and many other countries. This is where the mind is taken, under hypnosis, back to a time before the current body was born and asked to describe things that are happening around it. Depending on the hypnotist and the hypnotee the stories can be impressive in their accuracy and can be drawn out to encompass several different lifetimes in a single session. You really need a hypnotist who is at least sympathetic to Past Life Regression to achieve anything worthwhile though and you may have to search for a bit to find one who is. Incidentally, this is how many stage hypnotists get started when they pull Past Life Regression out as a 'party-piece' once they tell people, "I'm a hypnotist".

As for what hypnosis should not be used for… Well there's very little actually. Certainly treating even mild mental disorders is best left to psychiatric and psychology professionals. Even experienced therapy hypnotists would shy away from treating these problems as it may be all too easy to trigger an episode which, for the most part, therapists are not trained to cope with.

Many other subjects can be handled competently even by inexperienced hypnotists and I can really only reiterate that if you have an idea for something you think could be treated with hypnosis then discuss it with a hypnotist or two and see if they can come up with some ideas to help you.

Chapter 6 – Self Hypnosis

I'm going to stick my neck out a bit here and say to you that what you may think of as self hypnosis is not really what you are getting.

To many people self hypnosis is when you stick on a pair of headphones and listen to a recording which takes you into a hypnotic trance before guiding you through a self improvement routine of some kind – probably the usual quit smoking or lose weight sort of thing. To my way of thinking (and there are many more who think the same), this is still guided (hetero) hypnosis and no different to sitting yourself in front of a live hypnotist and listening to his voice guiding you through the self same routines. You merely have the advantage of being able to utilise the session at a time and place convenient to you.

Self hypnosis is when you talk yourself into a light trance and tell yourself what you want to happen. It seems difficult initially as you have to keep enough conscious thought available to talk to your unconscious mind, which seems a bit of a contradiction but it can be done and as with many things, gets easier with practice.

If you think of a sportsman getting himself 'into the zone' before springing into action, then you have an idea of what you can do. A mental rehearsal of the action they are about to perform is often the prelude to the successful completion of that action. The golfer's practice swing, the hurdler's leg action before the race, or even a high jumper's hand actions imitating the jump he is about to make are more than just muscle warming exercises, they are there to ensure the body knows what is required of it and even if the coach that encourages this behaviour doesn't call it self-hypnosis, in many ways it still is.

So to perform self-hypnosis, much of what happens is not different to what a hypnotist in a therapy situation would tell you to do.

Prepare the idea that you are going to use on yourself. This idea should be:

- Simple. A single sentence of less than a dozen words.
- Be framed in the positive – say "I am a non-smoker" rather than "I don't want to smoke any more".
- Be unambiguous. "I don't want to smoke any more" could be taken to read that "I don't want to smoke any less"!
- Use the present tense as if your wish has already happened or ensure you specify a specific time limit. "I will weigh 65kgs by Christmas 2012"

Your preparation should consist of the following steps:

- Write it a few times on a piece of paper to ensure it makes sense to you and to ingrain it into your memory.
- Switch off your phone and be sure you won't be disturbed for a while. 10 to 15 minutes is usually enough initially.
- Lie or sit down and make yourself as comfortable as possible. Kick off your shoes, loosen tight clothing. Close your eyes.
- Start at one end of your body, head or feet, it doesn't really matter, and tell yourself to relax that part of your body – and do so!
- Work your way up or down your body, relaxing each part as you go until you reach the 'other end'. This is to get you physically relaxed.

In your imagination, slowly walk down some stairs or through a peaceful wood or by a sea shore, whatever takes your fancy until you are totally mentally relaxed. Put as much detail in as you wish, the whole idea is to distract your mind from the here and now for a while. Stairs are a favourite of many as you go 'down' into trance, then you can ascend the stairs to emerge again.

- With your last piece of conscious attention, repeat your message to yourself a few times. It doesn't have to be out loud, but you should not read it off the paper, it should be in your head already. This is the biggest advantage to keeping it short and simple.

- Take a minute or so to absorb what you have said to yourself. Timing is not exact so there is no need to get a stopwatch out or set an alarm.
- In your imagination, reverse the path you just walked or climb back up the stairs.
- As you reach your destination point, put some animation into your thoughts, speed up your mental pace and tell yourself that you feel fit and healthy and ready to face the world again.

Finish by saying "One, two, three. Wide awake, I feel great" or something similar and positive, then open your eyes on 'three'.

Look at a clock or watch at this point and see how long that had taken you. If it was significantly different to the time you set aside, remind yourself to slow down or speed up a little as required – the former is more likely as we spend less time relaxing than we should. If you repeat this practice fairly often, you will get to the stage where you will be able to dictate to yourself beforehand how long you wish to spend and be accurate in your wish. At least one hypnotist I know is so good at this that he does not need an alarm clock and can wake up at whatever time he wishes no matter what time he goes to bed. So turn this self hypnosis routine into a pre-sleep routine with your suggestion to yourself being to sleep for 8 hours (or whatever) and become your own alarm clock.

This sort of self-hypnosis becomes much easier with practice and over time your suggestions could become a little more complex or become multiple suggestions in a single session. However, simple is best and it would be far better to do one session - one suggestion and do multiple sessions with yourself over a period of time of perhaps several hours rather than pile a load up for your unconscious mind to deal with all at once.

Chapter 7 – The Ideal hypnotee

So now you've read through this book, you know as much as you need to be able to go and see a hypnotist for a therapy session, to respond well to the hypnotist's suggestions and gain the maximum benefit for yourself from those suggestions. You know that if you go and see a stage hypnotist that you could go and be the ideal subject for him and perhaps be his top performer, participating in his set piece grand-finale, a place usually reserved for the people who respond the best to his suggestions.

You could also become an ambassador for this misunderstood group – the hypnotists, both the therapists and entertainers, who have to struggle through the public's perceptions of the media's usually uninformed mis-information, since you now know the truth of what really goes on and how the myths 'myth-inform' the outside world.

Who knows? You may now even get the idea to become a hypnotist yourself. To take some live courses, study some video lessons, read some books and join the elite group, helping others to cure their phobias or making them laugh and applaud at your show night after night. You will certainly find that the more you study, the more there is to study. Going down the therapy route will take you towards Neuro Linguistic Programming (NLP), Cognitive Behaviour

Therapy (CBT), Emotional Freedom Technique (EFT) and many other similar modalities. Looking into stage hypnosis will almost certainly have you looking at improvisational acting, stand-up comedy and stage craft.

Whatever you do, do it because you enjoy it. If you can get pleasure from what you do you can almost certainly pass on your enthusiasm to others and that makes it far easier for them to respond positively to you. Win-win all round.

About the author:

A man of many hats in his time, Steven Lucas has been (and still is, much of the following list) a simulator technician, an I.T. support technician, a flooring salesman, an internet marketer, a guitarist, bassist and drummer as well as an avid consumer of information, usually in the form of reading, both in paper books and electronic formats. He now feels that it's time to give some of that knowledge and experience back.

Although Steven has been interested in hypnosis since an early age he didn't really get really into it until he saw a stage hypnotist perform in Ibiza whilst he was on holiday. On Steven's return he started to look up hypnosis on the internet and found out some of the best names to study and promptly began to investigate their works. Steven now operates as a hypnosis-based therapist in the north Somerset area using the website http://www.yourmindtherapy.co.uk and performs on stage as SteeRange – The Reality Technician (have a Stee-Range experience) - http://www.steerange.com

Other works by Steven Lucas:

Web Site Management for the NEW WebSite Owner –
Web site management advice for someone who has to take
over looking after an established website including changing
pictures and layout, improving internal SEO and making life
easier for the new web master. Available from
http://www.wsmftnwso.com in pdf format, with some
valuable bonuses. The eBook is also available in Kindle
format on Amazon (USA, UK & Europe) without the bonuses
but at a lower cost. Search for Website Management. I'm
working on the other eBook formats.

Steven's hypnotherapist website:
http://www.yourmindtherapy.co.uk for hypnosis based
therapy in the south west corner of the UK

Steven's entertainment hypnosis website:
http://www.steerange.com

Steven's medical information website: http://www.know-
all.info – A website full of all sorts of information on all sorts
of subjects.

www.ingramcontent.com/pod-product-compliance
Lightning Source LLC
Chambersburg PA
CBHW060012300526
45794CB00003B/1176

* 9 7 8 1 4 7 9 2 3 1 3 8 6 *